PLUGGED IN ON PORN – GUIDE TO BREAKING THE BAD HABITS OF PORNOGRAPHY AND MASTURBATION

BY

TONY SAYERS

ABOUT THE AUTHOR

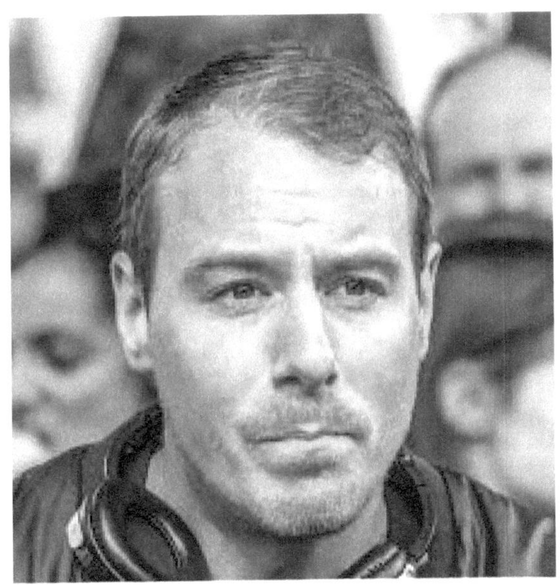

Tony Sayers is a passionate activist, vlogger, writer, and public speaker who in 2013 started to become aware of the deeper goings-on within this World and the hidden hands that control it. Since having these realisations he has been relentless in his work to expose the levels of corruption in society in an attempt to help others open their eyes. He is driven by doing what he can in his own way to help future generations enjoy a better World. His work has been mainly focused on human psychology, mind control, and spiritual laws. He is now progressing into technological, metaphysical manipulations, and energy healing work.

Born in Southend on Sea, Essex, UK he enjoyed a good childhood, although he found school quite challenging with other students and somewhat boring. His questioning of what is 'normal' had subconsciously already begun. From school, Tony went traveling when he was 21 which was a huge learning curve where he felt he got a real education observing how other cultures lived, and the vast differences between the developed and non-developed World. He also traveled to Nepal and researched Buddhism, which at the time which was to sew a spiritual seed in him that was to germinate later in life. After this period he went on to work in many standard jobs in both the Banking and Estate Agency Worlds, but never truly felt fulfilled, and feeling as if he was just going through the motions of life. It was in this period where he was so downbeat in the rigorous daily grind he started to ask the big questions in life which ultimately led him to these greater understandings about himself and the World, the learning is still going on today.

Sometimes controversial Tony is raw in how he expresses himself and his truth but is always coming from a place of care and desire for positive change. Tony has appeared on radio shows and spoke publicly which can be found on YouTube. He has his own website which is http://www.transcendingtimes.org where all his work can be found. To Subscribe To subscribe to his free weekly newsletter which has blogs, vlogs, media announcements and information on up and coming books just join here https://transcendingtimes.org/subscribe-to-newsletters/

Tony has authored other books including 'Are You Living Or Just

Existing?'and 'Ten Life Hacks To Beat The Matrix' both of which are available on Amazon.

www.transcendingtimes.org

INTRODUCTION

So I have to say writing a book on masturbation was not on my bucket list growing up, but the irony is breaking the bad habit of masturbation and porn has actually helped me achieve many of the goals and dreams I aspire to. I have really only been practicing abstention for around two years now, Being interested in all kinds of alternative health and therapies I had looked at the lot. Distilled water, urine therapy, plant-based diets, and fasting were among months and years spent in attempting to tune into a higher level of health and wellbeing, I was, and still am to some extent, obsessed with finding hacks to become the best version of myself.

There are so many benefits to abstention, many of which I will talk about in this book, that now it has literally become part of who I am as a person. I feel it has helped me on so many levels physically, emotionally, mentally, and certainly spiritually, and that going back now would just be like dancing with the devil again.

I tend to really trust my intuition and when I stumbled across a video on YouTube explaining how masturbation and in particular pornography is causing more damage to us than we realise, the penny almost dropped instantly. The issue is so multifaceted as I will go into, that it is vitally important that this subject is bought out into the open and looked at in a mature way, if you open your mind to this then you really do start to see not only the common sense in it but the science behind it also (I'm not talking about mainstream science here by the way who just spout whatever the systems wants) I'm talking about hundreds and thousands of testimonials of men practicing this everyday.

First-hand accounts are now all over the internet of how refraining from masturbation and holding onto your seed elevates you into hugely improving your life. That is not to say it is easy, far from it and there are times you feel like throwing in the towel. But ultimately if you give this a chance it will make you become a better man, and can be used as a very important tool in propelling you forward onto your life's purpose and becoming who you TRULY are.

We are living in such interesting times right now, and many men are starting to rise and step into a more authentic version of masculinity and authenticity. Many of us now want to evolve to something better than what we are showing up as. There is a real need for men to step into their innate power in these changing times.

We are surrounded by corruption and turmoil on many levels of society, and it really has been allowed to happen because there has been little to no resistance. Much of this has to fall on the shoulders of men, as our natural essence is that of protector, action taker, and really to be the cradle of protection for the females and innocents of society. We have been sold a false sense of masculinity with bravado, fake confidence, and this macho image. But where has this got us really? That is the question we have to ask ourselves.

Practicing abstination and breaking the bad habits of masturbation and pornography addiction is a massive step forward in not only respecting ourselves but respecting others. We are then leading by example and reconnecting with the true warrior within.

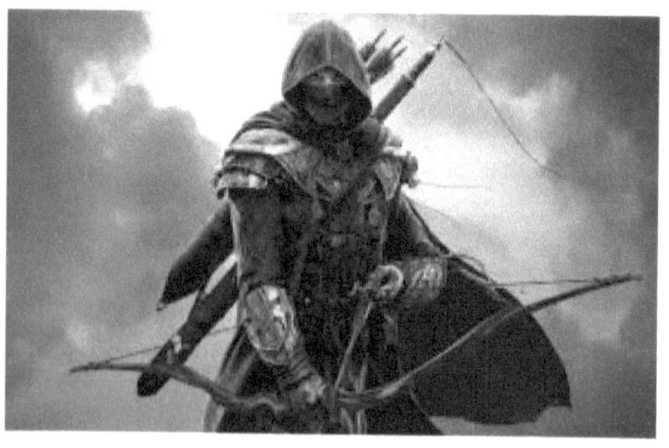

CONTENTS

THE SEXUALISATION OF SOCIETY

So really when you think about it everything starts here. To get to the reasons as to why men masturbate we must go to the root cause and look at our surroundings. There can be little doubt that we are surrounded by sex, half-naked women on billboards, newspapers, and almost every aspect of society. Music videos, movies, and TV programs are littered with sexual innuendoes, and with pornography freely available and generally unregulated, you can get whatever your fix is at a touch of a button.

Sex sells and the social conditioners of society know this only too well. Promiscuity is being encouraged more and more to the younger generations, and with 'role models' such as Rhinna releasing music about sadomasochism the screw is being turned ever more tightly towards a full-on sexual society. The reasons for this is for another book altogether, let's just say the movers and shakers of this World have a very perverted and sick view of where they want society to go. I talk about this issue extensively in my book 'Are You Living Or Just Existing?' Also available on Amazon. We really need to be asking WHY society is like this in the first place.

So with sex constantly being shoved in our faces is it any wonder that many men develop a craving for constant sexual gratification? I mean let's face it we have a part of our body that quite often will do the thinking for us! That is, of course, if we do not have any discipline.

As men, we have grown up to see

women as objects, just something we can stick our member in and then onto the next one. I grew up with it, and I admit I was like all my other mates. If you slept with a woman then it was considered a 'notch on the bedpost' and you were given a pat on the back by your friends. We have been indoctrinated to see this as normal, maybe it even hides our own insecurities in that sleeping with a woman could be considered to give you a nice little confidence boost.

One of the fundamental problems seems to be is that we have disrespected the feminine for so long we have forgotten what she stands for. She is the essence of creativity, nurture, care, and love. She is your mother, daughter, sister, or niece.

Funny how we forget those things when we are consumed by sexual thoughts. We must rediscover these qualities of the feminine. Yes physically women are absolutely beautiful, but us men make ourselves look ugly when we disrespect and just objectify her.

One thing often said within this community and something that I can vouch for myself is that once you have masturbated a feeling of guilt arises within you. Its almost as if subconsciously you know jacking off to a woman in an inauthentic way like that is wrong. It doesn't make you feel good at all. In fact when you consider the length of a male orgasm its barely worth the sock you do it in! (If that's how you do it!)

Could it be that at a subconscious level we know we are casting a shadow over women by doing this? Lack of respect? Or is it more what we have done to ourselves by doing the deed? We will get into this later on in the book but I would definitely say its a combination of both.

We cannot totally blame the social engineers of society as we all have free will to make our own choices. The amount of men who are even starting to question the act of masturbation is really encouraging. Man of these men are young maybe late teens or early twenties. They are already getting at a very young age that something is wrong with all this, and that actually it is causing harm to their personal progress and evolution

A sexual society can only remain as such if we buy into it. As men we have a responsibility to protect the feminine so she feels safe, we are there to supposedly stand up for the innocent, young, and exploited. Yet we have become the ones that do the exploiting ourselves. We can make all the excuses we want, we can say that we are 'wired this way' or that its 'just testosterone' but to me, we can all evolve to something greater than what we are, both individually and collectively. Those that want to stay stuck can keep those belief systems, however for the rest of us surely its time to take control of our lives, and then the World, and move it in the direction that we want it to go rather than the social engineers in government, media, and Hollywood. It is only with our acquiescence can this reality continue in such a way.

The way I see it is that we are the last generation of men who can make a change before a full-blown sexual society breaks out. I strongly feel that when you abstain from masturbation you are showing that you have both respect for yourself and for others. You're not just 'doing what others do' and in your own small way you're making a stand, thats without all the other benefits that we will go into.

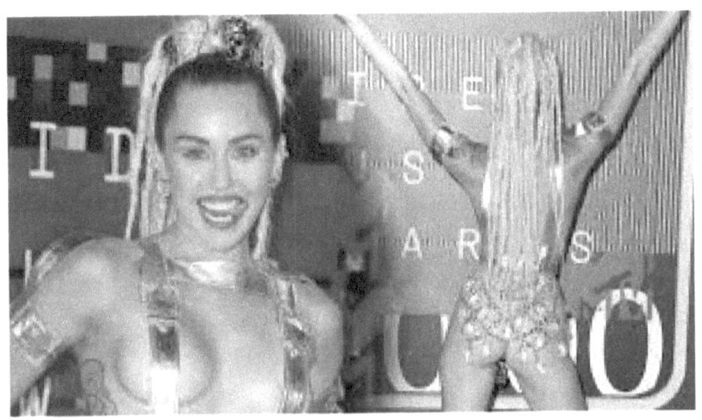

With any problems, a solution can only be found when we address the root cause of WHY something is happening, and this 24/7 bombardment of sex onto the human psyche stands as one of the biggest. On my own journey, I have rediscovered what sex really should be about and that is between two people who are in love, sex without love means nothing really, its just a quick bang and a bit of carnal gratification. Sex with your hand even less so!

Its not easy don't get me wrong and nobodies perfect, but we must acknowledge and recognise that part of this habit or addiction is down to the society around us, and that we have a choice to either stay as part of the problem, which will affect our children or grandchildren, or step up to the plate and become part of the solution.

Rejecting porn and the objectification of women will go along way towards developing a new respect for the feminine. This isn't some warped 'new wave feminist' viewpoint either, it's just me being brutally honest with how men view the opposite sex. I know because I used to be like that myself to an extent.

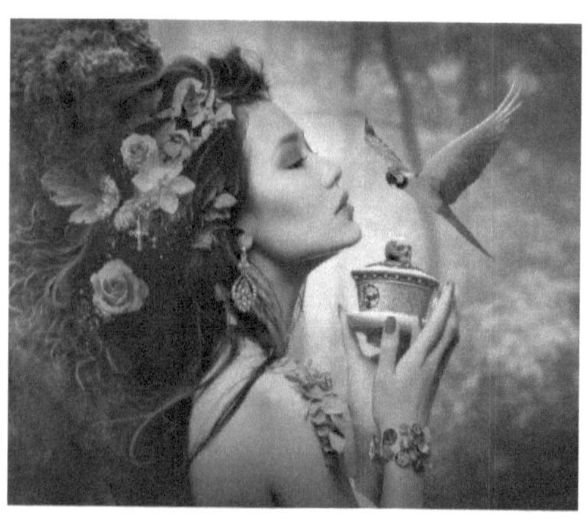

THE WHY BEHIND

There can be little doubt that when we masturbate it is mainly to make ourselves feel better, to get that little dopamine hit when we ejaculate so for a few seconds at least we forget about our problems. When you look at any addiction there is always something going on behind the scenes, something is hidden deep in the subconscious mind which is driving the need to self-harm, whether that be drugs, alcohol, food, or even masturbation it does not matter.

See advising people to just stop masturbating would be doing an injustice to you all, because there are many people doing that right now, many people are singing the benefits from the rooftops and rightly so, but they are not giving the root cause as to WHY any attention at all. So effectively you may stop masturbating but then you might start overeating or smoking for example.

The firefighter who tries to put out the flames of your pain with addictions will just turn his hose somewhere else unless we go deeper. The hard truth is we all have emotional wounds and traumas running through us from when we were children, some worse than others. Different kinds of abuse, betrayal and abandonment wounds, even if we had a decent childhood we still probably had to deal with stuff from school and just plain unconscious parenting.

All of these trials and tribulations stay with us into adulthood unless we do the hard, gut-wrenching, emotional work nobody wants to do! This particularly applies to men who generally run to the hills when it comes to facing their emotions. We have been sold a fake version of masculinity based around hiding our feelings and acting macho, which in reality is highly destructive as we are just walking around with wounds projecting our pain onto the World and onto others.

To stop masturbation is only a tiny piece of the puzzle and I really want to make that point crystal clear, you will find another vice if you don't go deep into yourself. Abstention will perhaps give you more inner strength and willpower to do that but you have to face the dark night of the soul if you TRULY want to become the best version of yourself.

I speak from first-hand experience with this, I had a decent childhood by most peoples standards, but there were events in my past that I had spent years either unconscious of or justifying to myself that 'there were a lot more people worse off than me'. Of course, this is true but your shit is still your shit so to speak. It still affects your behavior, relationships, and life in general.

Another problem is that society is set up to keep us looking outside of ourselves for healing and happiness. Think about it, gyms are like churches these days, but where are all the people queuing up at their local psychotherapist's office? Its all about how you look on the outside in today's society, huge importance is put on wearing the best clothes, having the right physical body, and getting the perfect 'selfie' look. We live in an ever-increasing narcissistic society. It breeds shallowness and from there soulless people whos only care in life is to look good.

Happiness is an inside job, no relationship, habit, or venture over to the otherside of the World will heal your inner turmoil, only you can do that yourself. It will follow you around and infect every aspect of your life both consciously and subconsciously until you go to where you do not want to go.

To go through this process is the hardest yet at the same time the most rewarding challenge a person can face. I am living proof, and although I am by no means the finished article, I am massively different than how I used to be. I no longer have the same fears and insecurities, I attract better quality people and circumstances into my life now. I function better in intimate relationships, I am no longer projecting my pain out on other people or myself.

This inner child work played such a huge part in my transformation that I decided I wanted to learn how to do it and help others which I am now so grateful I can. I am working with a lot of men right now to help heal the subconscious parts that drive them towards bad habits in the first place. You can contact me through my website www.transcendingtimes.org if you feel like this is something you would like to explore further.

I wouldn't suggest emotional healing as a 'should do' I would say its absolutely essential in moving towards becoming a more authentic version of you, and really getting at the root cause of the need to masturbate and any other habits that you may have to deal with. Otherwise, all you are doing is pouring buckets of water over the flames when you actually need a big firehose to put them all out!

STANDING WITH GREATS

So if you take on the challenge of abstention then you stand next to some great names throughout history, like me you may or may not resonate with what they do or what they stand for but it certainly seems many of those who have achieved something throughout history also applied the same principle of holding onto their seed.

Its not only famous people though, the number of online testimonials of a new generation of men who are smashing through goals, breaking barriers, and stepping into their power is all there for people to see at a fingertip. These men, some of which document their whole abstention journey go from shy and retiring, to confident and assured.

Muhammed Ali, Mike Tyson, and Manny Pacquiao would reportedly abstain from sex and masturbation months before a fight. Miles Davis famously said he didn't masturbate since it 'sapped your energy'. He said he'd fight Muhammad Ali if he 'masturbated before the fight'. David Haye the British boxer said 'I don't ejaculate 6 weeks before the fight. No sex, no masturbation, no nothing. It releases too much tension. It releases a lot of minerals and nutrients that your body needs and it releases them cheaply'

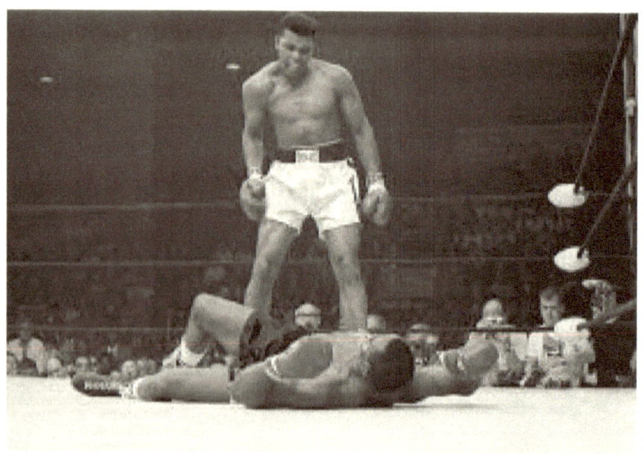

Friedrich Nietzsche the famous German philosopher said 'The reabsorption of semen by the blood is the strongest nourishment, and perhaps more than any other factor, it prompts the stimulus of power'. The Dali Lama, Winston Churchill, and Mark Twain are all said to be practitioners of abstention. So it really does go completely across the board in terms of sectors of society, and if its good enough for some of those names then its good enough for me!

Perhaps one of the greatest names to be linked with abstaining from masturbation is the great scientist Nicola Tesla, he was said to be completely celibate his whole life. He managed to create many inventions around free energy and essentially discovered how light can be harnessed and distributed. Of course, you won't learn about him at school because God forbid the power brokers of this World would hate you to find out that they are sitting on all of this technology. its too inconvenient for them to give us free energy, especially when the politicians and governments around the World are getting their palms literally greased with money from the fossil fuel industries! But hey that's for another book, but it is all easily researchable.

Nicola Tesla could quite possibly be one of the greatest minds to walk this planet. A true genius and to get through what he got through in a lifetime there was definitely some kind of superpower going on, or perhaps maybe he just wasn't throwing away his seed!

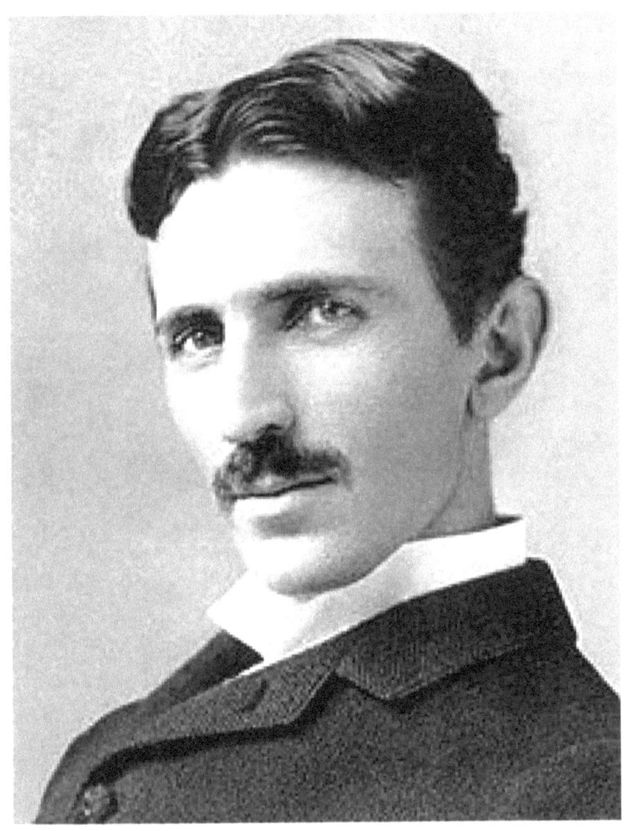

Tesla said on the subject 'The knowledge of how the mental and vital energy transform into what we want and achieve control over all feelings' There are many other names throughout history, writers, philosophers, and musicians all saying the same thing, some take it to higher extremes than others, yet the message is the same exercise your will in this area of life and you will reap the rewards.

THE SECRET TO SUCCESS

So why did all these greats live their lives in this way? Is it any coincidence that those who abstain from masturbation come to light up the World in their own unique ways? For me, that answer is very simple when you think about what you are losing when you masturbate.

For those 2 or 3 seconds of enjoyment you are literally throwing away your life force energy, you are throwing away what is essentially a substance that can create another human being. There is MASSIVE power in that. You are losing your very creative essence. So when you hold onto that you get to use it for you!

That essence can make you stronger, more focused, creative, and much more purpose-driven, which stands to reason as it has your very own DNA encoded within. Imagine what you feel like after you ejaculate, tired and lazy, not much motivation, maybe even a little ashamed and depressed. Well, imagine feeling the exact opposite of that all of the time.

I can not tell you what a difference this has had on me in my own life. I would go as far as to say it gives me maybe another 25-30% every day. I get things done, I'm up early in the morning, and I don't wake up tired and lethargic either. Mostly I start my days at 6am and finish as late as 12pm not feeling tired or weak.

As a creative person, the number of ideas and insights I get compared to when I used to regularly masturbate are on completely different levels now. Things flow like they have never flowed before, and I know that is massively down to holding onto my creative seed to use it for my own life.

Another huge difference I notice now is my general confidence has increased, I am much more comfortable in my own skin, and people seem to react differently to

me. Its like they can feel a different kind of energy you are omitting, its very subtle and we will explore this more shortly but it is definitely noticeable, and something many other people also report.

I will go more into the physical benefits later on but there is a noticeable difference in performance when I don't masturbate whatever the physical activity might be. I can run for longer, faster, lift more weights, and my recovery time is also decent (considering Im knocking on the door of the big 40 now!).

After the times I relapse (and we all do sometimes) that lethargy comes back, My mind seems slower and I feel less creative. I can almost border on the irritable, and sometimes feel a bit down. I liken it to the old Mario computer game when he headbutts the boxes and grows bigger. That's how I feel on nofap, and after a relapse, I feel like small Mario again.

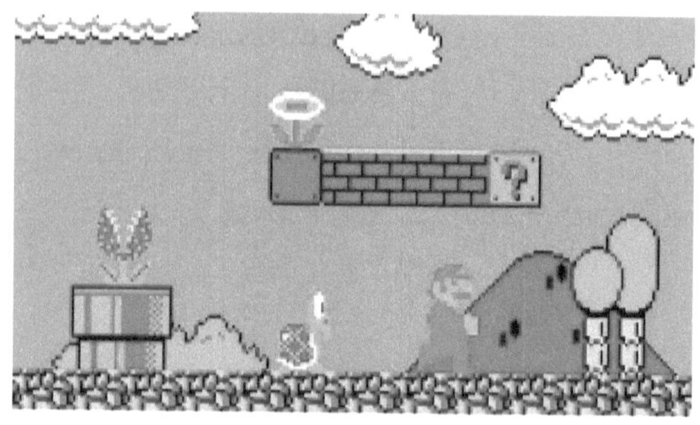

As I mentioned briefly earlier I definitely feel like practicing abstention helps you find your purpose in life, I was quite lucky in that I found what I was supposed to be doing about five years ago, however what abstention has done is refine that, it has helped me make better decisions and execute them in a much faster timescale.

It's like you have access to an extra pool of wisdom which knows what is best for you.

It's really encouraging to hear young guys who document their experience on YouTube talk about how confused and lacking in direction they were when they used to watch porn and masturbate. How they would feel lost and even bored, but how refraining has given them a new lease of life and a clear vision of where they are going.

You can see it in their faces from day 5 they look a mere shadow of what they look like and how they come across on say day 100! Full of life, energy, drive, and mission. Stepping into their true power, and what I would suggest is a more authentic type of masculinity.

I guess one of the most beautiful

positive offshoot effects of abstention is a new found respect for women, you no longer see them as objects and as something just to be used as gratification. You start to really appreciate the real beauty both internally and externally of women. How we need women to feel safe from this distorted and toxic view we have of them. They need us to step up as men so they can shine their love and nurturing energy onto this World which is of such desperate need of that right now. They will rebirth a much better reality here but we must hold space for them to do that. Nofap will help you rediscover your authentic love and respect for women which has always been there its just been lost in this over-sexualised society.

Not only will you have more respect for women but you will have more respect for yourself, you will develop the willpower to help in other aspects of your life. Maybe you might then go on to clean up your diet, get fit, or do some emotional healing.

Abstention will give you the strength to do all that, you will grow to love yourself a whole lot more. It's not the key to all your problems for sure but it makes things a whole lot easier to handle. You will generally just respect everyone a whole lot more. Self-love and self-respect mean that you can share that with others around you. People will notice the change in you, you will become a shining light in this World and your light is needed.

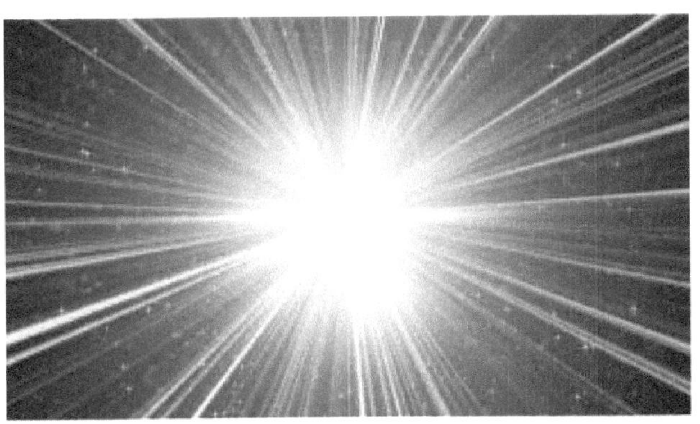

TONY SAYERS

THE SCIENCE BEHIND

So how exactly does this all work? What is it that makes the magic happen? Well a big part of it is that your semen has many different types of minerals, nutrients, and proteins some of which include vitamin c, calcium, magnesium, b12, nitrogen, and zinc. amongst others. Semen is actually only 1% sperm, the rest is made up of all this good stuff.

So common sense tells you that when you masturbate, especially if you do it regularly, then you're going to lose all these vital ingredients. This is the reason why lethargy and tiredness kick in after you ejaculate because you've literally just blown all of that out of your body for a 3-second hit of dopamine.

The issue is that with dopamine and

serotonin being the 'feel good' triggers of any addiction, the more you do it the more hits you're going to have, and the more you will feel the urge to masturbate. This is seen with any addiction alcoholism, drugs, even eating or shopping. Its all about getting those hits that take you away from whatever internal issue is going on with you at the time.

Looking back I distinctly remember masturbating when I had some drama or chaos going on in my life. You relate it to making you feel good, albeit very temporarily. As I mentioned in the second chapter, to get to the root cause of any addiction its important for us to go to the source of what drives it in the first place, even though it's probably the last thing that we want to do. Because ultimately you may give up masturbation but another addiction might kick in to replace this one as you have still not dealt with your emotional wounds and traumas.

With abstention in time, these nutrients and minerals are absorbed into the bloodstream which of course then has positive impacts on our physical body and how it functions. I have mentioned the physical benefits, but I can also say my skin is clearer when I refrain and my hair seems to be a little thicker too.

Increased energy and testosterone levels. After just one week without masturbation, your brain raises testosterone levels by up to 45% it is said, this could be perhaps why so many weightlifters experience being able to lift more weights refraining. I have also certainly found this to be the case.

Mental Clarity or reduced brain fog. Most people report a massive increase in memory and cognitive function. For example, being able to make a story flow, the ability to stay focused during a conversation or when you are working at your job/college, and making better choices based on consequences.

Evidence suggests that the longer you can go without masturbating the better the results. I always say though that semen retention should be just one tool in progressing as a man and a human being. What is your diet like? How fit are you? What emotional work are you doing? Are you too stressed? It's not a fix-all solution but it makes it a lot easier to then tackle other areas of your life. Practicing this will exercise your willpower probably more than anything else you have ever tried in your life as easy as it sounds (we've not touched on the hard bits yet!). This strengthening of the willpower will then help you drop other bad habits. Again there is science behind this.

When we have any addiction we

create neural pathways in the brain they then tend to just work on autopilot, I guess you could compare it to being on autopilot or just having a part of us that is automated. So with pornography addiction what you have done over the years is create these very deep neural pathways that are in a routine of telling you to look at porn. What refraining does is over time it rewires these neural pathways to fire in another way for you. A way in which it is at best not an addiction, and at worst something you are able to keep more under control. So essentially you are reprogramming yourself not to masturbate.

Not only is it reported to rewire the brain, but there are also many reports of it helping sexual dysfunction in men. Many have reported after practicing abstention for a period of time a better and stronger erection, others have reported being able to transcend premature ejaculation. The theory behind this is that over time the muscles and blood vessels in the penis get weaker due to continuous masturbation so it stands to reason that by stopping they will restrengthen again.

Other people have reported aches and pains they've had for years going away. Again this would make sense if you are holding onto your life-giving seed and keeping all those nutrients, it would give the body a chance to make use of those and heal on deeper levels.

When you're continuously getting dopamine and serotonin hits through masturbation you're then starved of those 'feel good' chemicals in your daily life. This is why many people who practice nofap also list better moods, and prolonged happiness as some of the major benefits. Again this is something I can vouch for myself.

Despite hundreds if not thousands of positive testimonials online from men who are practicing nofap mainstream 'science' has taken a more negative stance on the issue, even proposing that abstaining from masturbation can cause prostate cancer.

For me I don't trust mainstream science as far as I can throw it, much of it filtered down and repeated from people who serve a system which seeks to control and disempower people. Call me a conspiracy theorist but having a large population of men realigning with their power is not something the system wants.

I mean they might actually start standing up for things that matter in the World like illegal wars, tax evasion from the World's elite, and many other injustices and lies coming from those in power. It's much easier for them to control and dominate the population with men operating at a much lesser capability.

There are many benefits out there

that we are told are not good for us and visa versa. It always amazes me how the likes of McDonalds, Coca-Cola, and various alcoholic beverages are advertised at such length, particularly at sporting events like World Cups and Olympics. If they are so concerned about our health why are we not seeing avocados, bananas, smoothie recipes, and organic food being shoved in our faces in the same way?

According to mainstream science, we still don't have a cure for cancer when there are actually many people healing themselves already with products that have been banned by our governments?? So I don't think our health is at the top of their priority list to be honest. These subjects are detailed in my other book 'Are You Living Or Just Existing?' which really fleshes out the reasons as to why things are the way they are. So I would urge everyone to do their own research before deciding on anything rather than just taking what the mainstream authorities says at face value, that also includes questioning what I am saying!

TONY SAYERS

THE PROCESS

You now know the why and what for's so how to start and what to expect? Abstention is really separated into two categories 'hard mode' which refrains from all forms of PMO (porn, masturbation, and orgasm) and 'normal mode' which is no porn or masturbation, however, orgasm is acceptable. This is the version that men in relationships may prefer and I will offer yet another variation to this later on in the book which I practice myself.

Everyone has different levels of need and variations as to what is best for them. There are some dealing with very strong compulsions, and confusion caused by the imagery of porn. So they may seek to try to promote the fastest results with least temptations by cutting out everything during their reboot.

Others may just have a passing interest in the benefits of refraining and want to explore to see if it works for them. People have varying levels of commitment and need for this and its ok to explore it at your own pace. However, if you really want to experience what I have outlined in this book then the hard mode is the way you're going to get them.

For some going 'cold turkey' may be a step too far, in the beginning, there is no hard or fast rule. You might just want to give it a weeks trial or two weeks and then work it out from there. If you can get to two weeks without a relapse then that will boost your confidence and perhaps your desire to go longer, like I say it depends on your level of addiction or habit. Always listen to your own intuition and inner guidance, nobody can tell you exactly how long to go for or when to stop, it really needs to be something you decide for yourself. Some people are able to go hard mode and maintain this for many months even years, others it's a bit more stop- start and a case of working their way up.

My own advice would be to push yourself but be sensible about the goals you set for yourself. These things are definitely not easy but you have to strike a balance certainly in the beginning.

I liken this process to doing a detox or fast. When you first start you might go for a 7 day fast or something slightly shorter, then once you have conquered that you move onto a longer one, maybe a 14 days detox or 28 days. All the time you're also building up your willpower and inner strength to push the boundaries further. Of course, this isn't to say you shouldn't go cold turkey, I'm simply saying that you know yourself better than anyone else and you just need to tune into that.

There really is no failure with this, attempting to improve yourself in any which way should be viewed as a success. Ultimately what you're doing by abstaining is something that 99% of the World's population of men will never even attempt! But I want you to take this forward and implement this in the months and years to come because only then will you tap into this pool of life force energy which was once not available to you. This untapped energy has the potential to catapult your life in a way you never thought could be possible. If you need to start with smaller timeframes to build yourself up then so be it.

For me now it is a way of life, it doesn't even cross my mind to throw my life force energy away. I've lost count of how many months its been, and I have a girlfriend which I will explain later on! When I was transitioning away from this habit I could notice such a huge difference in my whole being from when I masturbated to when I didn't that it's just not worth it. It's just not worth giving up all that extra creativity, drive, energy, and power. So I simply don't. That is what I think the goal should be, to get far enough down the road with this that when you do relapse (and there is a very high chance you will) that the feeling of loss is so apparent to you that you really see the value in abstaining and that it doesn't have to be 'sold' to you by someone like me!

When going through this there will be times that you feel like bursting! Pent-up sexual energy, particularly if you masturbate a lot, can be a real problem, it will test your willpower like nothing else ever has. you will want to watch porn, have sex, and dream about the women like you have never done before! Sometimes in the early days, for me around day 30, you think you're going mad! All you want to do is have a release and it literally consumes your thoughts.

These times will test your resolve to the limits, it will really ask serious questions of you and how much you really want to push through. These periods are to be expected, and if you can approach them armed with solutions, you can also be overcome to make the situation more manageable.

There are many techniques people suggest for overcoming these times of massive temptations, some better than others. For me, I find that if I am feeling particularly horny then I will go out and exercise. See this pent-up sexual energy needs to be used, it needs to be recycled within the body somehow. Exercise is perfect for this, it circulates the energy and the horniness tends to leave. That's how you need to view this, in that this extra 25-30% now needs somewhere to go, it needs to be used for something. Now the benefits are two-fold here because not only are you holding onto your seed, you're harnessing the excess to work out and get fit! Choose an exercise you enjoy, there's no point going running if you hate running (like me). Make it fun then it doesn't have to feel like such a chore. Once you get a little down the line with this you will relish exercising, it has saved me from relapsing many times!

Another solution is to get creative, you now have all this creative energy at your disposal so use it! Write that book you always wanted to, or start that business you have always promised yourself you would. Channel this sexual drive into areas of your life that need attention it definitely works! The amount of testimonials from people who have gone on to achieve dreams and goals they have had for years is truly inspirational!

A quick solution if you are really on the edge of a relapse are cold showers, there are many benefits to cold showers anyway. On nofap they will stop you dead in your tracks if you think you're about to cave in, just run to the bathroom, whack the shower on full cold, and enjoy! You will hate them at first but after a while, you will see how they help you overcome uncontrollable desires.

These three are the best solutions I have discovered on my own journey, there are thousands of others out there which are easily researchable, you have to find your own coping mechanisms. The good thing is that the longer you stick with this, the same sexual desires tend to recede. They become much more under control, it's not that they go away, its just that you control them rather than them controlling you.

So what if you experience the dreaded

relapse? What if you tried all the techniques above and more but the temptation was just too much? First and foremost be kind to yourself, don't beat yourself up about it. You're human you attempted something and this is just a setback. Especially if you masturbated frequently before, coming off an addiction is never easy and the last thing you should do is give yourself a hard time.

At this point, I would delve deeper into why it happened. It's rarely just a moment of weakness, maybe in some people's opinion but I believe there is a why to everything we do. Were you feeling down or depressed about a certain situation? Often as I have said previously, we tend to masturbate for a quick dopamine hit to make us feel better.

Is there an unresolved issue that you have still not dealt with or that has not gone away? Are you unsatisfied with your job, a relationship, something that happened in the past? There is something there that you acted upon so just try to understand it and then take the necessary action to resolve the root cause.

Once you have analysed the situation and taken steps to resolve the why my advice would be to get back on the wagon again as soon as possible. Because what can tend to happen is that we get ourselves into negative mind loops, we think that 'I can't do this' or 'this is too hard' etc and that is the point where we often throw in the towel.

So I would say get back on the horse as soon as possible. Don't sit there and procrastinate and ponder the reasons as to why you can't do it. You CAN do it and deep down you know this too!

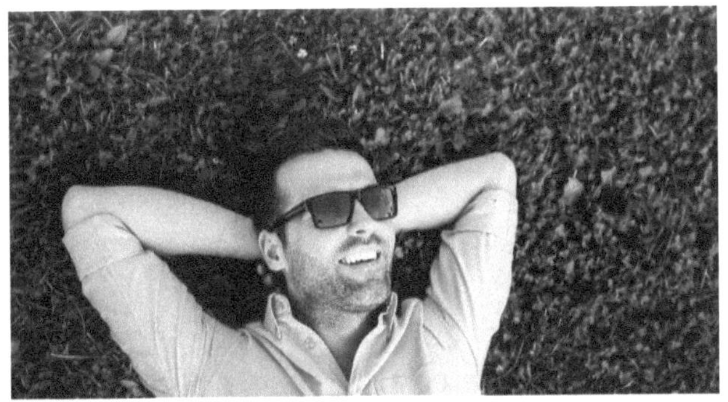

After a while, the inevitable 'flat line' will hit you. When this actually happens seems to vary from person to person from the research I have done. You can also have more than one, and this is highly likely the longer you practice nofap. For me, I had one at around 30 days then another around the 3-month mark.

So what is a flat line exactly? A flat line is actually viewed as something positive within the community, its an indication of the rewiring of the brain away from masturbation and pornography. It's your body's way of readjusting, but with that comes some temporary side effects that if you're not careful can throw you off course.

Symptoms include feeling lethargic, depressed, no energy, no motivation to do anything, and just downright, well flat! The research out there seems to indicate two main flatlines and then things get easier from there until you're totally rewired again. one is short term like mine after 30 days, and the other can be for a period of time afterward.

Again this can make you feel like giving up, and questioning is it all worth it? but in my experience, once you push through one of these flat lines then it's almost like you 'level up' again using the computer game analogy. You get your just rewards for pushing through and its all totally worth it in the end. Nothing good ever seems to come easy and this definitely applies to abstention so just try to ride it out if you can. They are inevitable and you need to be mentally prepared for them, just keep the end game in sight at all times!

ABSTENTION AND ATTRACTION

Let me start by saying this if you are interested in nofap purely to attract the opposite sex into your life then you're in it for the wrong reasons. This practice should be more about becoming the best version of yourself, discovering your purpose, and living your best life. It should be about moving away from objectifying women, and the negative spiritual connotations that come with that. Nofap should be about you ultimately growing and evolving into a better man and a better human.

There seems to be little doubt however that withholding your seed appears to have quite a profound effect on not just the opposite sex but people in general. This is where we get into the deeper layers of energy and how people can pick up on it.

When you hold onto your life force energy you are radiating outwards an energy most other men do not have because they generally all masturbate. It is fact that people, and in particular women, pick up on this energy. Many, many testimonials out there are providing more than enough evidence that this is the case.

Women have a natural subconscious sensor which is always looking for the best, strongest, and prime male as a mating partner, its just how they're wired. This is why they all flock to the football captain at school, or someone with a lot of power amongst his peers. Its simple law of the jungle, survival of the fittest stuff.

Women may not even be consciously aware that this even exists but it does. When you walk into a room and you're radiating at 25-30% higher in life force energy than your male counterparts then you can expect to be noticed.

Many testimonials report that women make more of an effort suddenly, smile more, and put themselves into the orbit of men that perhaps had no luck with women before. Because it boils simply down to the fact that the more life force you have, the more of a man you simply are, and that by default will attract more women into your life.

Also, it is possible it is a confidence issue as when refraining from masturbation after a period of time you will discover you are much more confident in your own skin. People report a huge improvement in social anxiety and it's my view that this is also reflected when you interact with others and in particular women. So essentially you have rediscovered yourself, and you are holding onto your life force energy which makes you very attractive to the opposite sex. I have experienced this on my own journey and its actually quite crazy the difference, it's like you have a secret weapon that only a few other men possess! As I say this is just one positive offshoot to many others in this process, and as fun as it is, really shouldn't be why you get involved with nofap in the first place.

It's not just women either, I find that I get a lot more respect from other men now too. It's almost like men can sense a difference in you that gets you almost immediate respect, and so it should because you have upped your game so to speak. You then have more power and control over what happens in both business and social situations. So this really does have positive effects in all other areas of your life.

ABSTENTION AND RELATIONSHIPS

So what about if you're in a relationship how can this work? Well there is a general consensus amongst the community that having sex with a partner and ejaculating is different than masturbating, and I guess is some ways it is. Certainly being in a loving relationship and ejaculating during sex is a lot better for you spiritually than masturbating over pornography, you're not buying into that bastardisation of the feminine for starters.

The habit of watching porn in a relationship can be damaging too, so cutting that side of it out will certainly help your relationship flourish from that angle, as there is no guilt or hiding anything (that is if you do hide it!) You're starving that pornography beast so that can only be a good thing.

I have full respect for any man that introduces this into their life when they're in a relationship, and there is definitely no right or wrong where this is concerned as it depends on you as a person and where you're at in life, and how far you actually want to take this.

For me even if I ejaculate during sex I really sense a loss in many aspects of my life. As I have discussed many of these benefits I have got used to now and have driven me on in life, yet I notice a large difference when I ejaculate even when having sex with my partner. There is a loss of abilities and energy that nothing else seems to give me.

So with that in mind, I now have sex without ejaculation, or others may even view it as some form of tantric. Even though I have never studied tantric I guess this is what it is. I can tell you now I have more pleasure having sex this way than the traditional. I feel a closeness to my partner, I don't want to just roll over afterward (as some of us men will relate to!) which obviously my partner prefers also!

I honestly have come to the conclusion that men are really only supposed to be ejaculating for procreation, that may sound extreme to some but is that just because we have been conditioned to believe that shooting our load regularly is just the done thing? As i have said before its actually encouraged.

This isn't speculation on my part, I have gone through this whole process. I have seen the differences, the evidence, and felt this power. I know for a fact that if I ejaculate, be it by myself or during sex with my partner I lose something, and for 3 seconds it's just not worth it. Apparently, there are other ways men can orgasm without actually ejaculating according to some tantric teachings which I have yet to explore. It goes without saying I have a very supportive girlfriend who is clued up on the deceptions at play in society and she gets it, probably 90% of other women would find it weird and that would be the end of it!

I'm not saying my way is the right way or indeed the only way, my only hope is for you to give this a go. To level up and experience some of which Tesla and Ali can testify to. To step into your true power, and using this life force, propel yourself onto your life purpose where ultimately you can then become the very best version of you with both a new found respect for the feminine and ultimately for yourself.

If you enjoyed this ebook please consider reviewing it on Amazon as it really does help me out!

For up to date details of my work, book launches, interviews, and talks please visit my website https://transcendingtimes.org/ and also consider subscribing to my weekly newsletter https://transcendingtimes.org/subscribe-to-newsletters/ for regular updates and free giveaways.

Both of my other books 'Are You Living Or Just Existing? and 'Ten Life Hacks To Beat The Matrix' are both available on Amazon.

To contact me or for session enquires please email me tony@transcendingtimes.org

www.ingramcontent.com/pod-product-compliance
Lightning Source LLC
Chambersburg PA
CBHW051225250726

48655CB00006B/2605